a guide to

yoga

Janice Jerusalim

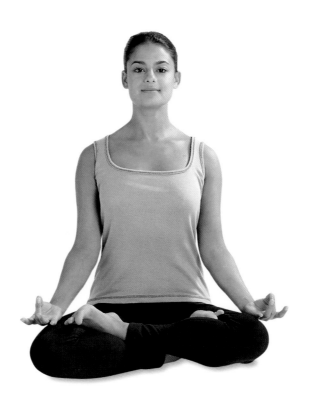

p

This is a Parragon Book

First published in 2002

Parragon

Queen Street House

4 Queen Street

Bath BA1 1HE

Copyright © Parragon 2002

This book was designed and produced by The Bridgewater Book Company.

ISBN: 0-75257-193-1

Printed in China

NOTE

Any information given in this book is not intended to taken as a replacement for medical

advice. Any person with a condition requiring medical attention should consult a qualified

medical practitioner or therapist before beginning any of the exercises in this book.

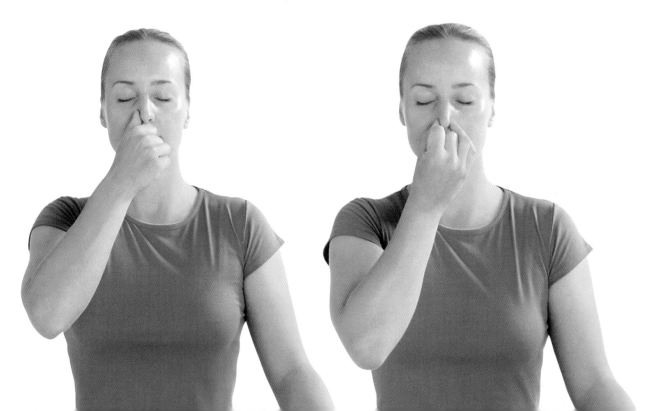

contents

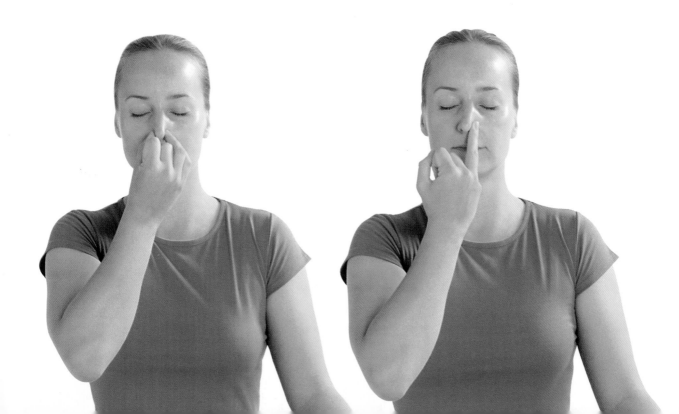

Introduction

If this little book for beginners inspires you to explore the system of yoga, it could become your first step towards the liberating journey of self-realisation. I took that step about 10 years ago, when I was ignorant of the philosophy and merely looking for a fitness programme that would increase my flexibility and improve my muscle tone.

I believe that I was very fortunate to have been introduced to Nasser, who was to become my yoga teacher for the following seven years. Through his gentle guidance it soon became apparent that the benefits of yoga far surpassed a physical fitness routine. He taught me that the mind and body are

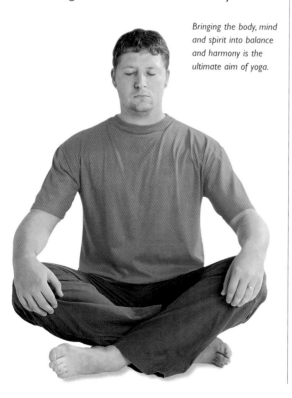

Bringing the body, mind and spirit into balance and harmony is the ultimate aim of yoga.

linked and that if the body is out of alignment, the mind cannot be in control. He taught me that stretching, purifying and healing the body would bring balance and harmony to the mind, thus creating health, happiness and fulfilment. I learned to let go of the negative conditioning of the past to become more conscious of how the emotional content of my thoughts today will determine my future reality.

I had been practising yoga with Nasser for about six years when he decided that I was ready to further my yoga practice with a trip to India. Arrangements were made for me to study at the Institute of Yogic Culture in Trivandrum, Kerala for a few weeks. Three hours of practice in the morning followed by a massage of the whole body (using the feet) and then a swim in the warm Indian Ocean was like being in paradise. Having trekked in the Himalayas a few years earlier I was already aware of how experiencing India can change your perceptions and affect you on a subtle level. However, I was unprepared for how

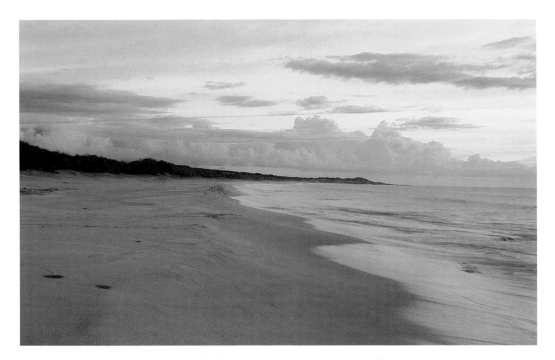

much this trip was to change my life. The physical exercises, the breathing techniques, the focus on the body, the massage and the beauty of Kerala opened me up to a new understanding of the principles of yoga. I returned to London, moved to a different area, changed my job, made new friends, started a new and very rewarding relationship and began to teach yoga in my spare time.

So what began as a simple quest for a fitness programme has led to a greater understanding of 'where I am coming from' and a much healthier lifestyle. I have yet to experience the true meaning of self-realisation, but I still have plenty of time to develop and yoga will continue to shape my present and create a positive future.

Yoga has been practised in India for thousands of years, and the stunning natural beauty of Kerala, above, makes it a fitting setting for this life-enhancing practice.

As we spiral off into the 'New Age of Aquarius', the energy around us is beginning to vibrate at a higher frequency. Time is speeding up and we need to find a way to calm down and slow down. There is unrest and turmoil in all parts of our planet and there has never been a more urgent time for us to restore the balance of nature and heal ourselves.

On a more 'down-to-earth' level, yoga is an easy, undemanding and enjoyable way of becoming healthier and stronger. All that is needed is a willingness to commit to positive change and to allow the many powerful benefits to start working through you.

Why yoga?

If you want to relax and become balanced, centred and calm, yoga will lead you there. If you want to achieve peace of mind and discover your hidden potential, yoga is the answer. Yoga will also help improve your physical health, tone your muscles and internal organs, relieve inner tension, reduce weight and strengthen your bones.

Yoga is for everyone

Forget about your fitness level. Forget about your age. Let go of your preconceived notions of what yoga is about. Yoga is for everyone. Yoga is a non-competitive, personal and enjoyable activity that can produce truly amazing results. You start at the beginning and you continue at your own pace. Whether you are a total beginner or an advanced practitioner, the benefits of yoga are many. With commitment, time and effort, yoga can change you as much or as little as you desire.

Yoga as art, science, and philosophy of life

The origins of yoga are shrouded in the mists of time. It is believed that the ancient wisdom known as 'the supreme science of life' was revealed to the great sages of ancient India three to four thousand years ago. This vast body of knowledge, when practised through the system of yoga, can lead to greater health, mental control and, ultimately, self-realisation.

Society today reflects the belief that disease, struggle and strife are natural to the human condition. Negative conditioning promotes ignorance, which prevents us from

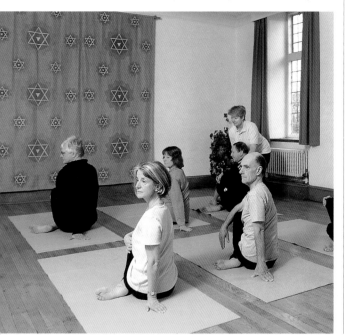

Practising in a class can aid your motivation but it is important to respect your own body and work at your own pace rather than comparing yourself to other students.

Oneness of all things

The word 'yoga' means 'union': union of mind, body and spirit – the union between us and the intelligent cosmic spirit of creation –'The Oneness of all Things'.

experiencing our true potential. These negative thoughts get stored in our bodies, causing blockages that disrupt the balance of health. The ageing of the body is largely an artificial process caused by stress, poor diet, ingestion of toxins and exposure to the harmful rays of the sun. By purifying the body and keeping it supple, we can reduce the process of cell deterioration.

Yoga provides a natural counter-balance to the stresses of modern life and can help you to achieve a sense of inner calm.

Yoga today

In our ever-changing world with its frenetic pace of life, technological advances and financial pressures, more and more of us are turning towards the principles of yoga. Recent scientific studies have shown that the regular practice of yoga decreases problems with breathing, digestion and blood pressure, eliminates stress and tension and helps people suffering with arthritis and arteriosclerosis. The results of a six-month study showed a dramatic increase in lung capacity, the ability to handle stress, and a reduction in body weight, cholesterol and blood-sugar levels.

Harmony and balance with hatha yoga

There are many forms of yoga, but hatha yoga is the one most commonly practised in the West. Hatha yoga concentrates on the physical body as the way towards self-realisation. It teaches us that gaining control over the body is the key to controlling the mind.

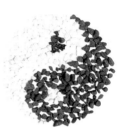

Yoga is a magical fitness programme that helps balance emotions, sharpen the intellect and bring peace of mind. The attention to the physical body with the emphasis on the postures is what makes this particular form of yoga so popular in our culture. You do not have to be spiritual to practise yoga. Start with the physical exercises – the postures – and see where they lead you. If you make the choice to practise regularly, not only will your body become more flexible, so will your mind. As we open our minds to the philosophy of yoga, we become open to life's possibilities. We learn to let go of the past and leave the baggage behind. Resistance will then break down so that new energy can flow into the empty spaces. Ultimately, with a little patience, discipline and practice, you will find yourself changing.

Practising the physical poses of yoga helps you to open up your body. Slowly, your mind will become more flexible and open too.

Ha (Sun) Tha (Moon)

Hatha yoga emphasises balancing the opposing forces in the body, such as masculine energy (the sun) and feminine energy (the moon), left and right, inhalation and exhalation, joy and sadness, and so on, thereby restoring the body to its natural equilibrium. Forward bends are followed by backward bends, standing postures by the inversions, contractions by expansions, and movements to the left by movements to the right.

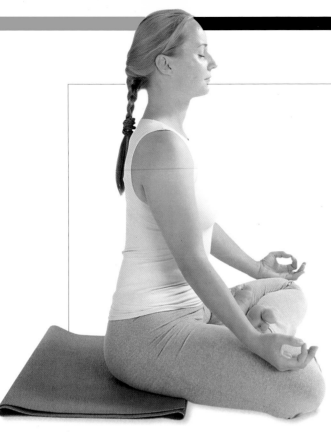

The five principles of yoga

3 Breath control – pranayama

Breathing techniques, or pranayama, increase the capacity of the lungs, enabling you to breath more fully. They help to strengthen the internal organs, improve mental control and deepen your ability to relax.

4 A nourishing diet

A well-balanced, nourishing diet will boost the immune system, ensure better health and help to calm the mind. As a result, your body will become more resistant to illness and disease and you will feel a greater sense of general well-being and health.

1 Relaxation

Rests your entire system and releases tension in the muscles. Exercise followed by relaxation dislodges blockages in the system and restores the body's normal energy flow. It helps to calm the mind.

5 Positive thinking and meditation

Yoga promotes positive thinking as one of its most important principles. It will train your mind to purify your thoughts so that a more confident you emerges. Meditation will ultimately lead to self-realisation – the real purpose of yoga.

2 Exercise – the asanas

The yoga postures (known as asanas) help to stretch and tone all the muscles and strengthen bones and ligaments. Asanas improve circulation and keep the spine, muscles and joints more flexible. They also help to relieve depression by increasing 'feel-good' endorphins in the body.

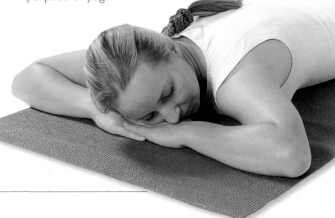

Making a commitment to a healthier lifestyle

The word 'commitment' implies discipline and finding the time to develop a regular practice. 'Yet another routine to fit into an already hectic lifestyle', you may say in despair. The very word 'commitment' can be off-putting. But wouldn't it be wonderful to devote some time to slow down, take a deep breath and let out all the tension?

Once you begin to realise the benefits of a system that not only promotes well-being but also reduces the accumulated stress of your working day, the discipline no longer seems such a chore. The mind will soon become accustomed to accepting yoga practice as a part of everyday life – a natural and enjoyable habit. Forget about the problem

Once you start to incorporate yoga into your daily life, it will quickly become an enjoyable and natural habit rather than a chore.

of finding the time. You will achieve more in each day when your mind is focused, your pulse is normal, your blood pressure is regulated, your muscles are more relaxed and your breathing patterns are steady. The more often you consciously allow yourself to become centred and balanced, the more empowered and successful you will become. You can't afford not to find the time. All that is then required is peace, quiet and commitment. It doesn't matter how out of shape or inflexible you may be to begin with, your increased vitality will definitely lighten the schedule of your day. Don't forget – your health and happiness are your responsibility.

Creating your own plan

Reading is an excellent start to finding out what yoga is about. The deeper your understanding of the yoga philosophy, the more you will be able to focus on how yoga can be of benefit to you. You can apply all you know to your own personalised programme. Over time, however, the best way to learn is with a teacher who can give you proper guidance, answer your questions and help you fine-tune the postures. You could begin by committing yourself to a class once a week, and then perhaps make a plan to practise one or two half-hour sessions at home. The most important objective is to practise regularly. Stick to a plan and soon the benefits will become obvious. Remember that yoga is not about guilt. Some yoga is better than no yoga. No two bodies are alike and no particular technique is suitable for everyone. You may need to experiment for a while with different styles of teaching until you find your own particular path.

Guidelines for practising yoga

● Start at the appropriate level and go at your own pace. Yoga is not about competition.

● A yoga session always requires a warm-up period. Your muscles need to become more fluid before attempting the complex stretches.

● Do not force yourself into the postures. Push yourself just to the 'edge' of the discomfort, breathe into the muscles involved and hold the position for a few breaths. With practice you will ease yourself deeper and deeper into the posture until one day – whoosh – the breakthrough will occur!

● Practise barefoot and in light, comfortable clothing.

● Don't practise on a full stomach. You will need to wait for up to four hours after a large meal, and two hours after a snack.

● Remove contact lenses and tie up long hair.

● If is is cold, work in a heated room. As you become more adept you will be able to generate your own body heat.

● Ideally the session should take place somewhere quiet and peaceful. To avoid unexpected interruptions, disconnect the telephone, turn off the mobile phone and remove your watch.

● Work on a non-slip mat that is long enough for your entire body to rest on comfortably.

From the unknown to the known

The Universal Mind choreographs everything that is happening with ultimate intelligence. It permeates every fibre of existence, and everything that is alive is an expression of this intelligence. Our bodies and all we perceive is the transformation of this consciousness from the unknown and invisible into the known and visible.

The process of creation is how Divinity expresses itself. The physical universe is pure consciousness (energy) in motion. When we see that our true nature is universal intelligence expressing itself, we begin to realise the unlimited potential of who and what we are.

What is prana?

Prana is the subtle force that animates all manifestations of creation. We extract this 'life current' from the oxygen we breathe and it then circulates throughout our bodies. By practising yoga, more prana is obtained and stored and one feels greater connection to the 'oneness of all things'.

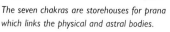

The seven chakras are storehouses for prana which links the physical and astral bodies.

The chakras and the nadis

According to the yogic sages, our physical body is encircled and interpenetrated by a subtle, astral body. Just as a physical body has nerves, the astral body has its counterparts, the nadis. There are 72,000 nadis – the sushumna, ida and pingala are most important.

The sushumna nadi corresponds to the spinal column; the ida nadi rises from the base of the spine through the trunk and ends in the left nostril; the pingala nadi rises from the base of the spine and ends in the right nostril. The ida and pingala nadis are said to criss-cross as they rise and the points at which they cross over are where the chakras are located.

The seven chakras of the astral body

There are seven main chakras (wheels of energy) in the astral body and many nadis come together here. Six chakras are found along the sushumna, which follows the spinal column, and the seventh is found at the crown. Chakras store prana; the energy becomes finer as it moves up from the base of the chakras to the crown.

Vishuddha or throat chakra

The fifth chakra, situated at the base of the skull, is linked to the glandular system and to expression. Blocked energy in this area creates difficulties with communication.

Manipura or solar plexus chakra

The third chakra, in the solar plexus area, draws in the yellow ray. It has to do with how we create balance within ourselves. Since it relates to the digestive system, it is an important centre for healing and the main store for prana.

Sahasrara or crown chakra

The crown chakra absorbs the violet ray and is the spiritual centre where true wisdom and understanding reside. Opening this chakra through meditation practices can – after much time and effort – lead to the ultimate goals of self-realisation and enlightenment.

Ajna or brow chakra

The sixth chakra is located between the eyebrows at the point known as the 'third eye'. It is associated with the colour indigo and it is in this chakra that conscious and unconscious knowledge meet. Opening the third eye and allowing universal energy to flow freely through it will put you in touch with your innate intuitive and psychic powers.

Swadhishtana or sexual chakra

This chakra is located just behind the genitals. It absorbs the orange ray and is concerned with our passions and sexuality. When we allow energy to flow freely here, this area of our lives will be positive. However, blocked energy can result in sexual or reproductive problems.

Muladhara or root chakra

At the base of the spine, this chakra draws in the red ray. It is concerned with our ability to survive and adapt and gives us stability. Too much or too little energy here can block us and make us afraid of change.

Yogic breathing

Yogic breathing, or pranayama, revitalises the entire body, balances the emotions and promotes clarity of mind. All the breathing exercises described here are performed sitting down, keeping the spine, neck and head in a straight line. This will facilitate the flow of prana and create the space for the lungs to expand more fully.

Full yogic breathing

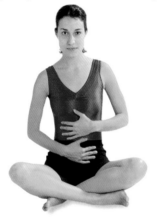

1

Sit cross-legged (sitting on a cushion relieves tension in the lower back and knees). Place one hand on the ribcage, the other on the abdomen. Keep your back straight, chin parallel to the floor and shoulders relaxed.

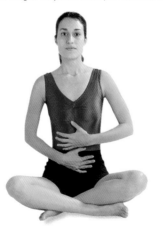

2

Make sure that you breathe through your nose with your mouth closed. Inhale slowly, feeling the abdomen expanding first, then the ribcage, and finally feel the air filling the entire chest area.

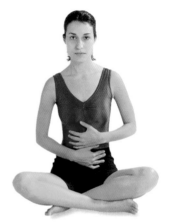

3

As you exhale, the air will leave the lower lungs first, then the ribcage area, and lastly the chest. Check that you fill your entire lungs with air and that your breathing is slow, rhythmic and deep.

Breathe for life

According to yogic belief, life expectancy is linked to the frequency of respiration. The tortoise, which is a reptile, breathes very slowly and lives a long life. A small mammal, such as a rat, breathes faster and has a much shorter life. If we can learn to slow down our breathing, yogis believe that we can add years onto our lives.

Ujjayi breathing – *the key to conscious breathing*

The main type of breathing practised is known as the ujjayi (pronounced ooh-jai-yee) breathing. In Sanskrit, *uj* means 'to expand' and *jayi* means 'success' – so we practise the ujjayi method of breathing 'to expand and flow into our success'. It is characterised by a soft, deep, almost hollow sound coming from the throat.

Ujjayi breathing is not difficult to learn. All you need to do is narrow the vocal chords slightly as you inhale through the nose with the mouth closed. As the breath passes through the restricted epiglottis, the breath will vibrate at the back of the throat. Slowly draw in long breaths. As you exhale you should hear a throaty sound. The narrowing of the valve in the throat will (once you have got the hang of it) help regulate the intake of oxygen and the throaty sound will bring your attention to the breathing process.

Benefits of ujjayi breathing

Ujjayi breathing cools the mind, soothes the nerves and strengthens the abdomen. It is a useful tool that can be used in all aspects of your daily life. It helps you to reduce stress, develop mindfulness and appreciate the beauty of life in all its detail.

Anuloma viloma – *alternate nostril breathing*

The benefit of practising this exercise is that it strengthens the whole respiratory system and rids the body of toxins that have built up through stress and pollution. Try to practise alternate nostril breathing every day.

1

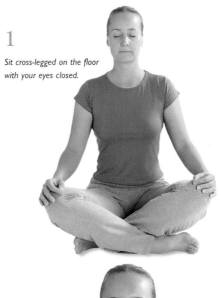

Sit cross-legged on the floor with your eyes closed.

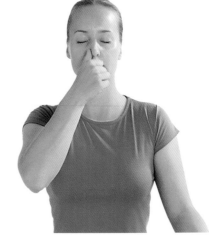

2

Close the right nostril with the right thumb and, slowly and smoothly, exhale through the left nostril for a count of four.

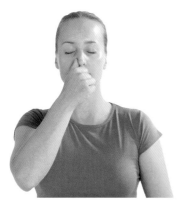

3

Continuing to keep the right nostril closed, inhale through the left nostril, again slowly and smoothly for a count of four. Stay centred and breathe slowly and deeply.

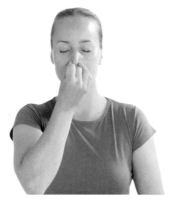

4

Close your left nostril with the third or ring finger of your right hand. Turn the first two fingers inwards to touch the base of the thumb.

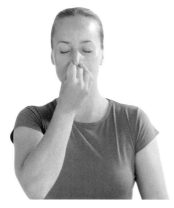

5

Continuing to keep both of your nostrils closed, retain your breath in your lungs for as long as you possibly can.

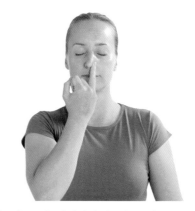

6

Release the right nostril and exhale slowly, with control, to a count of four.

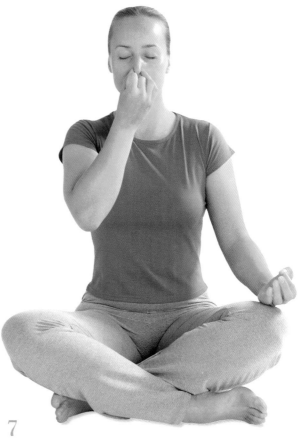

7

Inhale through the right nostril, use the thumb to close it, hold for a count of four, then exhale through the left nostril. This completes one round of alternate nostril breathing. Repeat this exercise 10 times.

Kapalabhati

Kapalabhati means 'skull shining' and its effects are to clear the mind. The forced exhalation rids the lower lungs of stale air, clearing space for fresh oxygen to cleanse the respiratory system. The movement of the diaphragm tones the stomach, heart and liver.

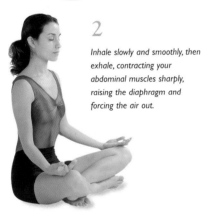

1

Sit up straight with your legs either crossed or in the half lotus position (see page 42). If you are naturally flexible, you can try this exercise in the full lotus position (see page 43).

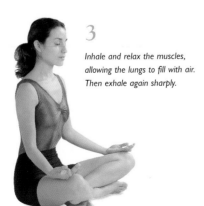

2

Inhale slowly and smoothly, then exhale, contracting your abdominal muscles sharply, raising the diaphragm and forcing the air out.

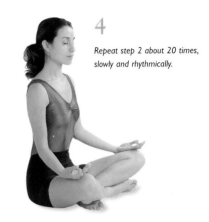

3

Inhale and relax the muscles, allowing the lungs to fill with air. Then exhale again sharply.

4

Repeat step 2 about 20 times, slowly and rhythmically.

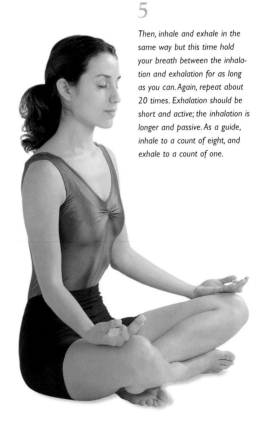

5

Then, inhale and exhale in the same way but this time hold your breath between the inhalation and exhalation for as long as you can. Again, repeat about 20 times. Exhalation should be short and active; the inhalation is longer and passive. As a guide, inhale to a count of eight, and exhale to a count of one.

Asanas

In yoga, the word asana means 'posture'. The movements are gentle and take into account the entire being. They form part of an psycho-physical system intended to awaken individuals to the experience of their full potential. Performed regularly, the postures have a profound effect in freeing a person from fear and conditioning.

Asanas are performed slowly and meditatively using deep abdominal breathing. They are designed to make the body strong enough to hold the positions for a sufficient period of time without discomfort. The real work occurs when you are holding the pose. The idea is to keep still while the position is maintained, to breathe consciously into the pose and to focus your attention on the rhythmic sound of your breathing. Body and mind will then naturally move into stillness and equilibrium. Once you are comfortable in a position, you can take yourself in deeper by stretching just a little further.

It has been said that there are as many yoga postures as there are creatures in the world, but of course it is only practical for us to concentrate on a few. Not only does the practice of yoga require you to mould your body into a particular pose (many of them mimic animals), it also asks you to identify with the qualities of the pose you are

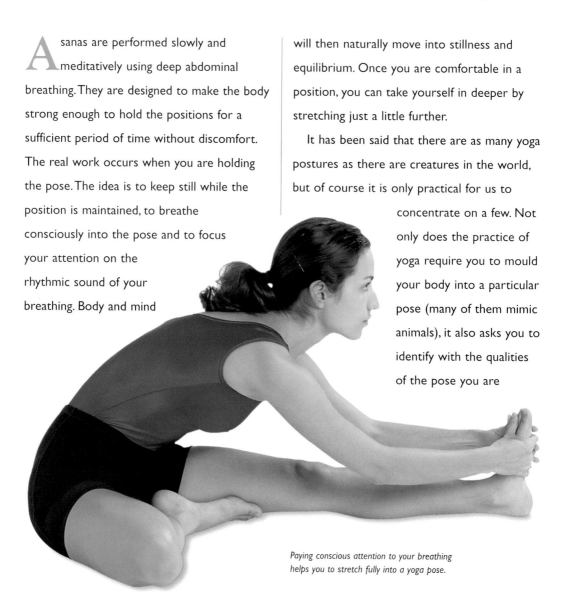

Paying conscious attention to your breathing helps you to stretch fully into a yoga pose.

performing. So for example, when you are performing the cat posture, you should feel yourself possessing the qualities of a cat as you move into the exercise; try to feel as you imagine a cat would feel; feel the arch of your back and the stretch of your spine.

Benefits of asanas

The various postures of a basic yoga session will stretch, strengthen and tone every muscle in the body, and there are many other benefits to be gained from the practice of asanas. Some postures will work on a particular organ of the body, while others will help regulate the endocrine system. The twisting, bending and stretching movements increase flexibility of the muscles and joints as well as massaging the internal organs and glands. They also improve the circulation, ensuring that a rich supply of nutrients and oxygen reach all the cells of the body. The most important work of the yoga asanas, however, is in strengthening and purifying the nervous system, especially the spinal cord and spinal nerves, because these correspond to the channels for prana in the astral body. The increase of pranic energy will help to awaken the spiritual potential.

The loss of vitality and the ill-health we suffer are caused by the running down of the body systems due to neglect, under-stimulation, laziness and unhealthy lifestyle.

The power of the mind

Before entering into a posture, visualise yourself performing it perfectly. Then, with focus and control, move into the pose.

Regular practice of the asanas will promote a state of mental well-being and physical health. The techniques are designed to maximise vitality and youthfulness, reduce stress, depression and hypertension, improve concentration and help balance the emotions.

When you start practising yoga, it will be the physical experience that will affect you. As you gradually develop and progress, you will begin to experience the sensation of pranic energy as it starts to flow more freely through the channels.

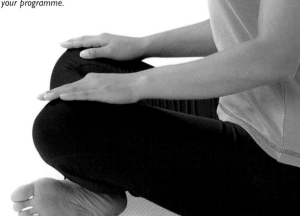

Start at the beginning: breathe slowly and allow yourself to build on the small, gradual changes you will notice as you persevere with your programme.

Mudra and mantra magic

Technically, mudras refer to a variety of yoga postures designed to prevent energy escaping from the body. They also refer to certain hand gestures performed during pranayama (see page 14) and meditation. The word 'mudra' means 'seal'.

Yoga mudra

This mudra is excellent for improving the functioning of the liver, spleen, kidneys, pancreas, bladder and uterus. The yoga mudra also helps to relieve constipation.

Caution

It is very important that you do not attempt this exercise if you are pregnant or suffering from any abdominal problem.

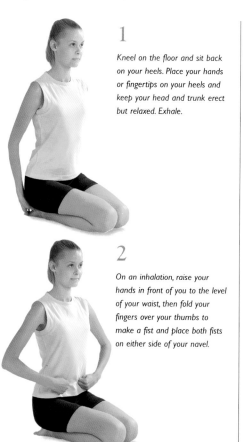

1
Kneel on the floor and sit back on your heels. Place your hands or fingertips on your heels and keep your head and trunk erect but relaxed. Exhale.

2
On an inhalation, raise your hands in front of you to the level of your waist, then fold your fingers over your thumbs to make a fist and place both fists on either side of your navel.

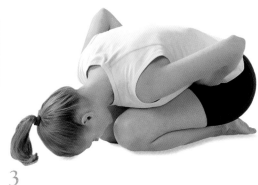

3
Exhale and then, keeping your buttocks on your heels, stretch your spine from your hips by slowly bringing your head towards the floor. Hold, with your forehead on the floor, and breathe for a minute, relaxing the abdomen. Come up and rest on your heels, palms on your thighs.

Attaining wisdom – Jnana mudra

Sit with your hands resting on your knees, palms facing upwards. Bring the left index finger to touch the middle of the left thumb, and the right index finger to the middle of the right thumb. This mudra opens one up to the beauty of life and promotes harmony.

Aswini mudra

Practising this mudra daily strengthens the pelvic muscles that control the bladder and rectum. It is an especially good exercise for women. Start with 30 seconds and build up to five minutes. You can kneel, stand or sit.

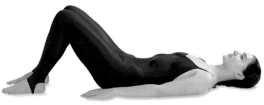

1

Lie on your back with your knees bent. Breathe rhythmically for about 20 seconds. Now contract the sphincter muscles (at the opening of your rectum), hold the tension for a count of five, breathing rhythmically while you do so, and then relax. Repeat six times. Women should simultaneously contract and relax the vaginal muscles.

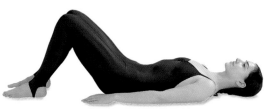

2

Pull the sphincter and all the pelvic floor muscles inwards and upwards. Hold the tension for a count of three, breathing rhythmically while you do so, and relax. Practise this exercise for up to half a minute in total.

The Divine Om mudra

Sit with your palms facing upwards, hands resting on the knees. Join the tip of the right thumb with the tip of the right index finger and repeat on your left. The two circles created represent the cycle of Divinity.

Mantras

Mantras are sounds that resonate in the body and evoke energy. The chanting of mantras calms the mind, awakens the senses and stimulates the chakras. Through repetition, mantras can help the mind on its quest towards enlightenment.

Yogic mantras

- The highest mantra of all is 'Om'. Yogis believe that this is the sound by which the universe was created. It means 'all that is' – infinity and eternity.

- The natural sound of the breath – SOHAM (pronounced SO-HAM) is also a mantra. It means 'I Am that I Am', signifying the Divine has no limits.

- OM NAMAH SIVAYA (pronounced OM NA-MAH SHE-VA YA) is a mantra that helps to conquer the ego, which blocks the pathway to self-fulfilment.

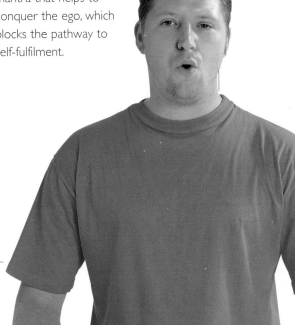

Let yourself go – relax

No matter where we live, today's world is stressful. We are bombarded with stimuli, perhaps pressured by money problems, insecure in our jobs, overworked, underpaid, controlled by the system, anxious about the future. You could say we are overloaded as we struggle to keep up with the pace of living in the 21st century.

As a result of all these pressures, we spend most of our time in a state of mental and physical tension. We clench our jaws, frown, hold our breath and tighten our muscles. The consistent contraction of our muscles drains our energy, causing fatigue. We suffer from bad backs, headaches, poor digestion, heart problems and a string of stress-related illnesses.

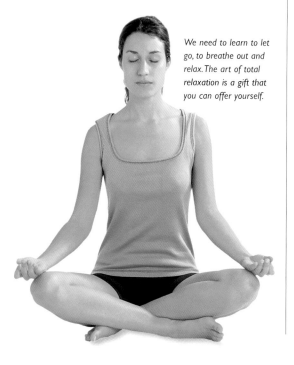

We need to learn to let go, to breathe out and relax. The art of total relaxation is a gift that you can offer yourself.

Relaxation is an essential part of yoga practice. Most people find it difficult to relax because they have never learned how to do it. To relax the body and focus the mind, you need to be either lying down or sitting up with your back and neck properly aligned. This allows the neuroelectrical system and the blood circulation to function efficiently.

Tension causes contraction of the muscles and contraction causes constriction, which leads to energy becoming blocked in the body. Once you consciously start to release the tension – the tightness, the holding on to protect yourself – you will begin to experience yourself expanding both mentally and physically. Relaxation is our natural state of being and the more familiar you become with being relaxed, the more it will spill out into your everyday life. You will start to become more aware of situations and circumstances that cause you to contract and close down and you will no longer wish to be at the mercy of your environment.

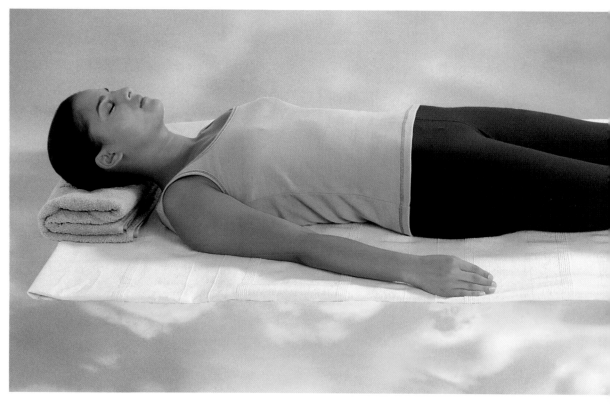

Once your body is relaxed, you need to relax your mind by letting go of all your preoccupations, fears, worries and anxieties through paying attention to your breath. Slower, deeper breathing will lead you to a calm and centred space. Allow yourself to let go, relax and enjoy the sensation of surrender.

As the body starts to relax, certain physiological changes will occur – the pulse rate will drop and tension will be released. Relaxation will bring mind and body into balance, reduce fatigue, release and expel toxins and revitalise the entire system. When you truly start to experience yourself in

Even when lying down, we can hold onto body tension. Make yourself as comfortable as possible – a folded towel under the head helps relieve tension in the neck – then simply allow the ground to support you.

stillness, you will feel calm and peaceful and you will begin to open up to a new awareness of who you really are. A few minutes of deep relaxation will be more effective in reducing tiredness than a whole night of restless sleep.

A yoga session should always begin with a period of relaxation. The body will also need to rest between postures to recover from the exertions of the exercise and to give the mind space to prepare for the next pose.

S a v a s a n a — t h e C o r p s e p o s e

This posture is one of the most important of all the asanas, for only when we truly learn to relax can we allow energy to flow freely through our body. Relaxing can be one of the most difficult poses for us to master. You just lie on the floor and relax. The essence of peace comes from within and the aim of Savasana is to relax the body so completely that the mind is set free and energy can flow freely.

The underlying purpose of yoga is to unite the self with the Absolute, to become conscious of 'I AM' in the infinite and eternal 'NOW', to achieve enlightenment. The Corpse pose teaches us to relax so completely that our bodies become irrelevant, like a corpse – dead – for it is only when we understand death that we begin to understand life. We need to turn our attention inwards because it is from within that the journey towards self-realisation begins. Master Savasana and you will have mastered your mind.

1

Make sure that you are warm enough. Lie down comfortably on your back and close your eyes.

2

Turn your legs in and out and then let them flop out to the sides. Your feet should be about 60 cm (2 ft) apart. Thighs, knees and toes are turned outwards. Turn your arms and let them fall out at a 45-degree angle to your body. Palms are upturned.

3

Turn your head gently from side to side and then return it to the centre. Make sure that you are lying symmetrically on the floor.

Find the inner quiet

Let yourself go, drop all the anxieties of the day and allow yourself to sink into the peaceful pool of your quiet mind. Learning how to relax both body and the mind deepens the beneficial effects of the asanas.

4

Relax your feet. Now, take your attention to your calves and feel them relax. Next, relax your thighs, then let your hips relax onto the floor. Work up to your buttocks, relax them, then your lower back, your abdomen, your middle and upper back and your chest. Relax your shoulders and feel the tension dropping out onto the floor. Then, relax your arms, hands and neck. Let your eyes relax into their sockets and feel your face muscles and scalp becoming soft and relaxed.

5

Mentally scan over your body for any tension; whenever you find a tense muscle, tighten it first, then relax it. Scan your awareness around and through your body, and be alert to any discomfort. Allow yourself to 'melt' into the floor.

6

Breathe into your abdomen and with each exhalation feel the weight of your body sinking deeper into the floor. Focus your attention by listening to the sound of your breath. Enjoy the sensation of the weight of your body being fully supported by the floor beneath you.

7

If your mind starts to wander, gently bring yourself back to stillness by concentrating on the slow rhythm of your breathing. The length of the inhalation, exhalation and the pause between them should be the same. The pause should follow the exhalation.

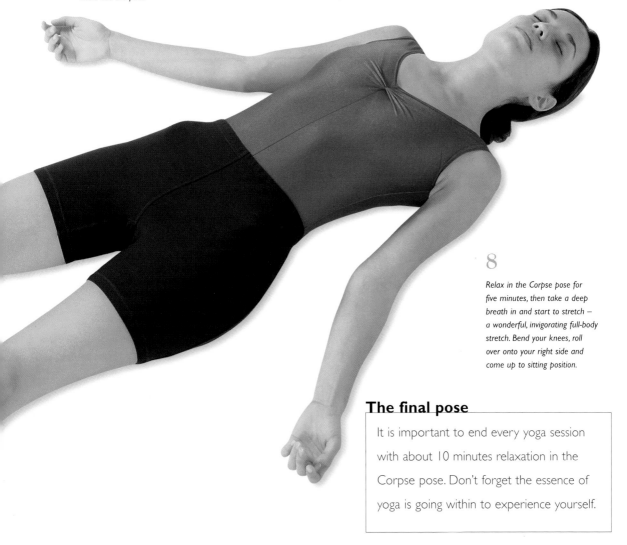

8

Relax in the Corpse pose for five minutes, then take a deep breath in and start to stretch – a wonderful, invigorating full-body stretch. Bend your knees, roll over onto your right side and come up to sitting position.

The final pose

It is important to end every yoga session with about 10 minutes relaxation in the Corpse pose. Don't forget the essence of yoga is going within to experience yourself.

Warming up

Before beginning any yoga programme, it is important to ease yourself into it by warming up the muscles and loosening the joints before moving onto the asanas.

Neck rolls

For this exercise you should sit cross-legged, with your back straight but relaxed. Rotating the neck slowly will help to release blocked energy in the neck, shoulders and upper back. Take care to work through the exercise slowly and gently, and stop if you feel any pain.

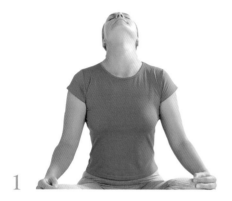

1

Hang your head forwards so that your chin rests on your chest for a few moments. Then, slowly drop your head back as far as you comfortably can and feel the stretch. Repeat this 5–6 times.

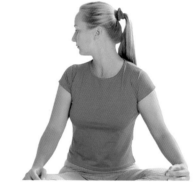

3

Turn your head slowly to look over your right shoulder. Look back as far as possible. Return to the centre and then turn your head to look over your left shoulder. Repeat this stretch 5–6 times.

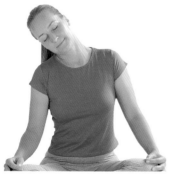

2

Now, take your right ear down to your right shoulder. Hold for a few moments. Bring your head back to the centre, then take your left ear down to your left shoulder. Return to the centre. Repeat on both sides.

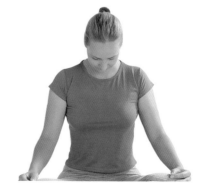

4

Drop your chin to your chest and then slowly rotate your head in a clockwise direction 2–3 times. Bring your head back to the centre and then gently rotate it anti-clockwise 2–3 times.

Shoulder rotation

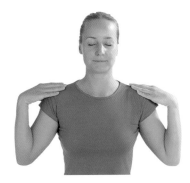

1

Sit cross-legged on the floor. Place both of your hands gently on your shoulders with your elbows pointing downwards.

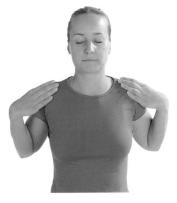

2

Inhale and slowly rotate your arms backwards, trying to close up your shoulder blades as you do this. Go only as far as feels comfortable.

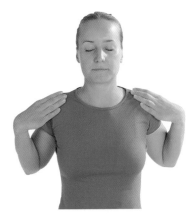

3

Exhale and bring your arms forward, making big rotations with your elbows. Repeat the movement eight times.

Leg stretches

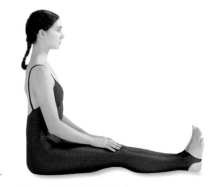

1

Sit on the floor with your legs stretched out in front of you, heels together.

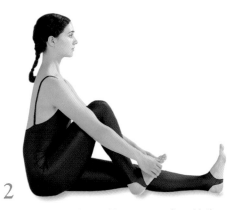

2

Gently bend the right knee and bring your arms forward (without tensing the shoulders). Take hold of your toes with both of your hands.

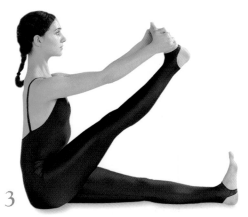

3

Straighten the leg and raise it up as far as possible. Bend the leg, relax and repeat. Change legs and repeat twice.

Bilikasana – *the Cat*

For this posture, visualise yourself as a cat arching and stretching its back.

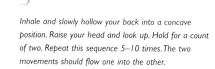

1

Kneel on all fours with your arms shoulder-width apart.

2

Exhale and arch your back up as high as possible. Keep your head between your arms and look towards your navel. Hold this pose for a count of two.

3

Inhale and slowly hollow your back into a concave position. Raise your head and look up. Hold for a count of two. Repeat this sequence 5–10 times. The two movements should flow one into the other.

Uttanasana – *Forward Extension*

This is an excellent posture for releasing the shoulders and stretching the hamstrings.

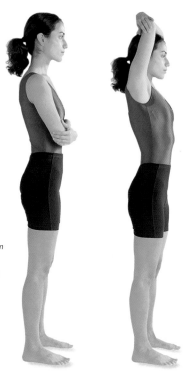

2

Inhale and take your arms up over your head, still holding your elbows. Draw your waist slightly back. Feel a strong stretch up through the back of your legs.

1

Stand with your feet about 30 cm (1 ft) apart. Exhale and catch hold of your elbows so that your right hand is holding your left elbow and vice versa.

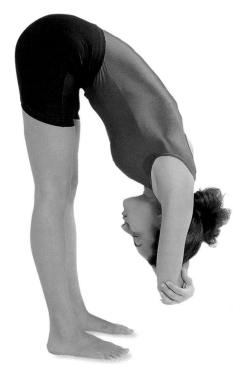

Tadasana – *Mountain pose*

This is the basic standing posture. It involves bringing the energies of body and mind into stillness and balance.

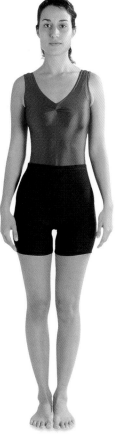

1

Stand with your feet together, your big toes and heels touching. Your arms should hang loosely by your sides, palms facing inwards.

2

Lift your body, extending upwards from the base of your spine. Your shoulders should be relaxed with your chest open. Look straight ahead.

3

Exhale and slowly bend downwards, bringing your arms as close to your chest as possible. Pull your elbows towards your body and down to bring your trunk as far down as possible. Now bring your hips further forward to keep your legs vertical.

3

Pull up your thigh muscles from your knees. Make sure that you are equally balanced and root your feet into the floor.

4

Keep your knees straight (but not locked) and your leg muscles pulled up. Relax your head. Blood will now rush to your head, nourishing your brain with nutrients. Remain in this position for about 30 seconds, remembering to breathe slowly and smoothly.

4

Using the ujjayi method of breathing (see page 15), take a few slow, rhythmic breaths. Remain focused and balanced.

Namaste mudra – *the Prayer position*

Place the palms together with the fingers extending upwards as in the prayer position. Now bring your hands to your heart as a gesture of peace and respect, and to honour the light within.

Surya namaskar – the Sun Salutations

This graceful sequence is done as one continuous movement to the rhythm of your breath. It is an excellent warming-up exercise.

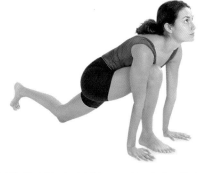

2

Inhale and stretch your arms up, with your hands open. Bend back from the waist, hips forwards.

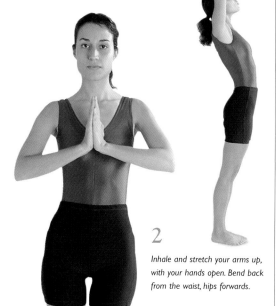

1

Stand in Tadasana (Mountain posture – see page 29) Take a few, deep ujjayi breaths (see page 15). Exhale and bring your hands together in Namaste, the prayer position (see page 29).

3

Exhale and bend forwards. Place your hands beside your feet. Bend your legs if you need to.

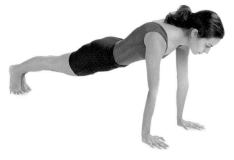

4

Inhale. Take the left leg back, left knee touching the floor. The hands and right leg are in front. Arch your back, lift your chin and look up.

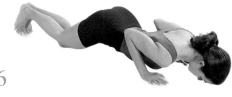

5

Retain your breath and take the right leg back. Support your weight on your hands and toes. The head, back and legs make a straight line.

6

As you exhale, lower your knees to the floor. Let your chest, then your forehead touch the floor. Your hands should be flat on the ground.

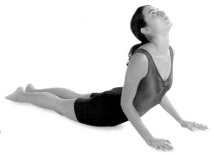

7

Inhale, lower the hips to floor and arch the spine back. Look up, tilting the head back. (This is Cobra pose – see pages 48–49).

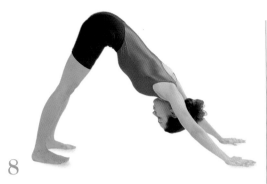

8

Exhale, roll your weight onto your feet and raise up the hips. Push your heels down and hang your head (Downward Dog pose – see page 34).

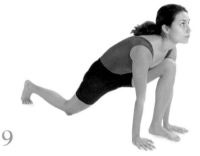

9

Inhale, step back with the right leg, right knee on floor. The left leg is in front, knee bent and foot flat. Look up and back (this 'mirrors' step 4).

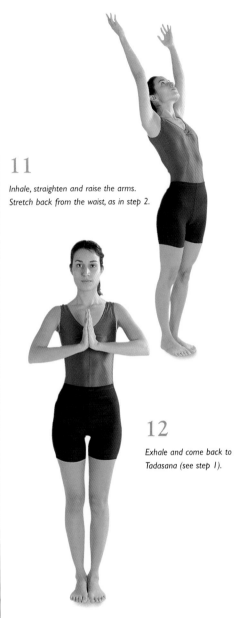

11

Inhale, straighten and raise the arms. Stretch back from the waist, as in step 2.

12

Exhale and come back to Tadasana (see step 1).

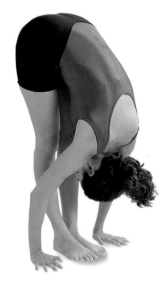

10

Exhale and, without moving your hands, move the back leg forwards, then bend down from the waist as in step 3.

Benefits of Sun Salutations

- Focuses and calms the mind

- Strengthens major organs and muscles

- Stimulates digestion

- Increases flexibility of the spine and joints

The standing postures

The standing postures are about developing strength, power and balance. They teach us how to stand with presence and self-assurance and how to remain centred in the moment. You will notice that the times you lose balance in these poses will be at times when your concentration wavers and you are no longer focused.

Pada Hasthasana – *the Standing Forward Bend*

'You are only as young as your spine.' This is an excellent pose for improving posture and promoting youthful vitality.

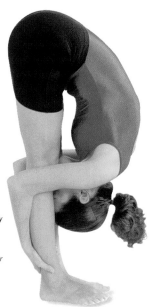

2

Exhale and bend forwards, catching the backs of your legs with your hands. Keep your body weight centred and your legs straight. Do not drop the hips. Take your forehead towards your legs. You may wish to extend further by taking hold of your big toes with your respective thumbs. Hold for five ujjayi breaths (see page 15), then inhale and straighten up slowly.

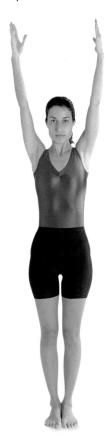

1

Stand with your legs together, the weight of your body on the balls of your feet. Inhale and stretch your arms above your head. Extend your body from the base of your spine to your fingertips. Pull up the muscles of your thighs from your kneecaps. Your hips should be pointing upwards and your knees straight.

Benefits of Pada Hasthasana

- Invigorates the nervous system
- Stretches muscles at the back of the legs
- Takes nourishing blood to the brain
- Lengthens the spine, improving suppleness and elasticity
- Tones muscles on the back of the body

Trikonasana – the Triangle Pose

This posture has many variations that can be learned once you have become more familiar with the basic practice. It involves an intense stretch all along the side of the body, from your feet to the tips of your fingers.

Benefits of Trikonasana

- A complete lateral stretch
- Tones spinal nerves and abdominal organs
- Improves digestion; stimulates circulation
- Reduces pain in the lower back

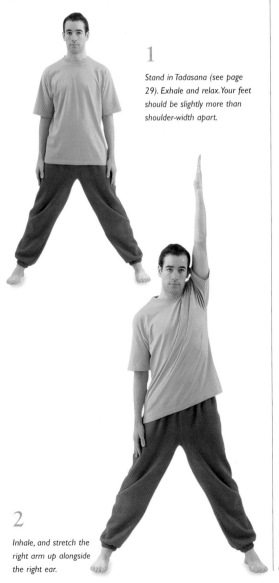
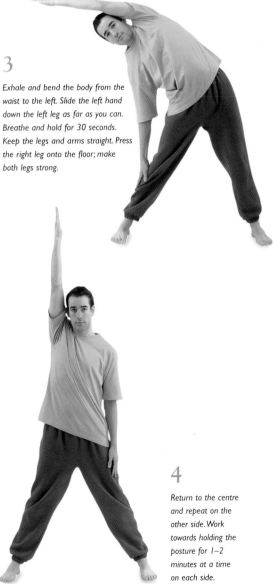

1

Stand in Tadasana (see page 29). Exhale and relax. Your feet should be slightly more than shoulder-width apart.

2

Inhale, and stretch the right arm up alongside the right ear.

3

Exhale and bend the body from the waist to the left. Slide the left hand down the left leg as far as you can. Breathe and hold for 30 seconds. Keep the legs and arms straight. Press the right leg onto the floor; make both legs strong.

4

Return to the centre and repeat on the other side. Work towards holding the posture for 1–2 minutes at a time on each side.

Adho Mukha Shvanasana – Downward-facing Dog

It doesn't take much imagination to visualise the way in which a dog stretches its spine when it first stands up after lying down for some time. This posture is one that most people will recognise as a classic yoga pose. The trick is to concentrate on lengthening and stretching out the lower back, rather than rounding the back. Remember to feel yourself as a dog stretching forwards. Besides stretching the spine and hamstrings, the Downward-facing Dog pose brings heat to the body and gives the heart a rest.

2

Lift up your tailbone and bring your knees off the floor so that your body forms an upside down 'V' shape. Your hands should be shoulder-width apart, fingers open, with your weight evenly distributed on your palms and all 10 fingers. Keep your arms straight.

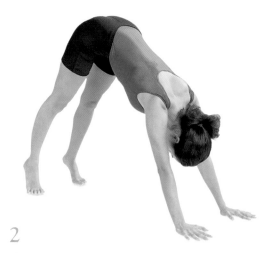

1

Go down to the floor on your hands and knees.

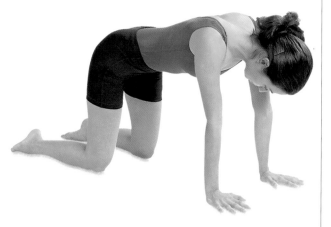

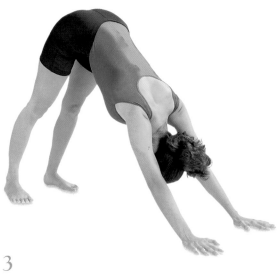

3

Now take your head between your arms and look to your navel. Point your hips upwards. Slowly take your heels to the floor and straighten your legs. Hold the position, taking five ujjayi breaths (see page 15).

4

If you have trouble getting your heels on the floor, try concentrating on the seated forward bends (see pages 36–39) to help loosen the backs of your legs first. Eventually you will master this posture and it will feel very relaxing, but it can seem quite hard work at first.

Parsvottanasana – *Extreme Sideways Stretch*

This is an excellent exercise for toning your abdomen, correcting drooping shoulders and developing flexibility of hips, spine, and wrists.

1

Stand in Tadasana (see page 29). Join the palms behind your back in the Prayer position (Namaste).

2

Inhale. Take the feet 1 m (3 ft) apart. Turn the left in 45 degrees and the right 90 degrees to the right. Turn trunk and hips to right; bend back from the tailbone.

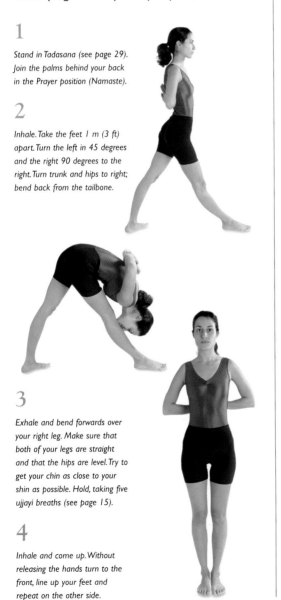

3

Exhale and bend forwards over your right leg. Make sure that both of your legs are straight and that the hips are level. Try to get your chin as close to your shin as possible. Hold, taking five ujjayi breaths (see page 15).

4

Inhale and come up. Without releasing the hands turn to the front, line up your feet and repeat on the other side.

Namaste – *the Prayer Position*

Join the palms behind the back, fingers upwards. Move the hands up between the shoulders, palms together and elbows and shoulders down.

Virabhadrasana – *the Warrior pose*

Think of the strength, balance and nobility of a warrior. Feel the power as your hands stretch up to the sun and your feet root to the earth.

1

Exhale and stand with your feet about 1–1.2 m (3–4 ft) apart. Turn your left foot inwards to the right about 45 degrees, and turn the right foot outwards about 90 degrees to the right. Bend the right leg and turn your body to the right. The left leg should be straight behind you.

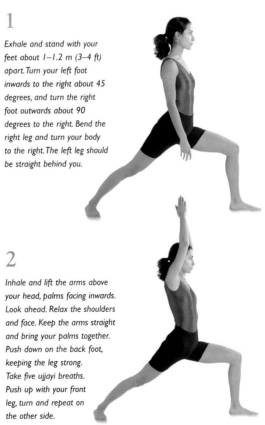

2

Inhale and lift the arms above your head, palms facing inwards. Look ahead. Relax the shoulders and face. Keep the arms straight and bring your palms together. Push down on the back foot, keeping the leg strong. Take five ujjayi breaths. Push up with your front leg, turn and repeat on the other side.

Focusing inwards with forward bends

The forward bends are excellent for helping you focus inwards – you bend forwards and your heart moves inwards. They are great for stretching out and loosening up the muscles in the lower back and for lengthening the hamstrings.

Paschimothanasana – the Forward Bend

This is a stretch all the way up the back of the body, from calves to thighs, along the spine and up to the head. It works to rejuvenate the system.

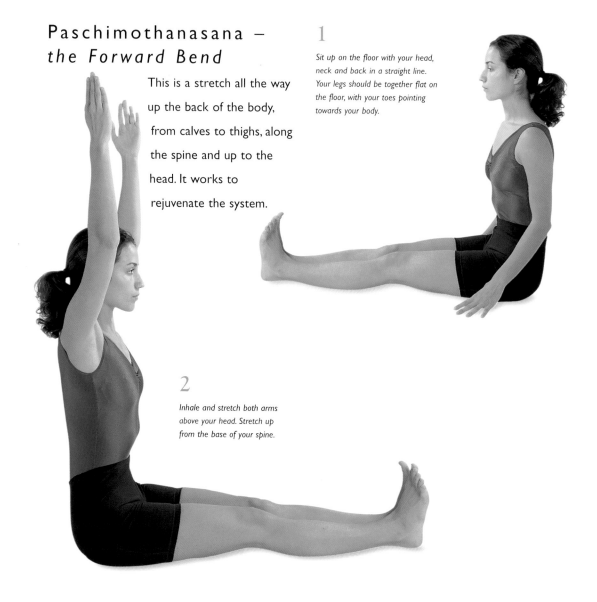

1

Sit up on the floor with your head, neck and back in a straight line. Your legs should be together flat on the floor, with your toes pointing towards your body.

2

Inhale and stretch both arms above your head. Stretch up from the base of your spine.

3

Exhale and bend forwards from your hips to catch hold of your feet, ankles or shins, whichever feels most comfortable to you. Inhale, and look upwards, moving your chin forwards and up. Keeping hold of your feet, lift your back up, stretching up through your spine and pushing forwards with your abdomen to avoid rounding your back.

Benefits of Paschimothanasana

- Stimulates and tones the digestive system, helping to counteract obesity, relieving constipation and regulating the pancreatic function

- Strengthens the hamstrings

- Increases the elasticity of the lower back

- Energises the nervous system

- Greatly improves ability to concentrate and focus the mind

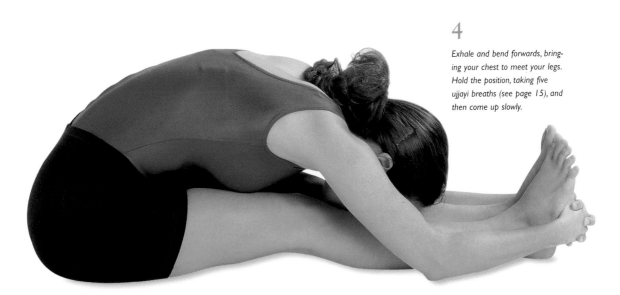

4

Exhale and bend forwards, bringing your chest to meet your legs. Hold the position, taking five ujjayi breaths (see page 15), and then come up slowly.

Janu Shirshasana – *Sitting One Leg pose*

The benefits of this posture are much the same as for the previous one (the Forward Bend). However, this position will also work on opening up the hips.

Tips

- Make sure that you bend forwards from the hips and not from the waist. This applies to all the forward-bending poses.

- Be patient with yourself if at first your body feels stiff and unyielding. With regular practice you will gradually start to stretch out and open up.

- Remember, yoga is not about the ego. Forget about being competitive.

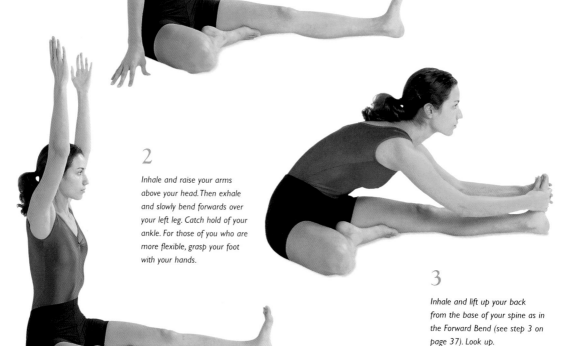

1

Bend your right leg and place the foot against the top of the left inner thigh. Your right knee should now be forming an angle of almost 90 degrees to your left leg. Sit on the floor with your left leg straight out in front of you and your toes pointing upwards.

2

Inhale and raise your arms above your head. Then exhale and slowly bend forwards over your left leg. Catch hold of your ankle. For those of you who are more flexible, grasp your foot with your hands.

3

Inhale and lift up your back from the base of your spine as in the Forward Bend (see step 3 on page 37). Look up.

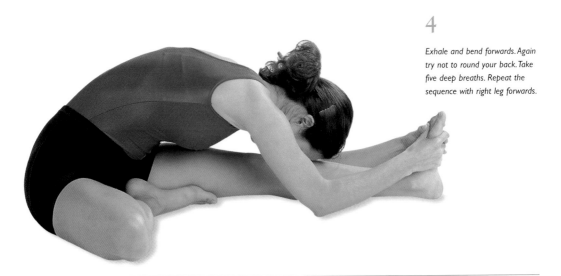

4

*Exhale and bend forwards. Again
try not to round your back. Take
five deep breaths. Repeat the
sequence with right leg forwards.*

Mudhasana – *the Pose of the Child*

This is a wonderful relaxing posture; it makes you feel safe and nurtured, as if you are back in the womb. It stimulates respiration, relieves lower back pain and releases tension in the shoulders. It is an excellent position for counterposing backward bends and for relaxing the body between postures.

1

*Kneel on the floor and sit back on your heels. Your buttocks should
touch your heels. Use a pillow between your buttocks and the backs of
your legs if it feels more comfortable.*

2

*Bend forwards, taking your forehead to the floor. Your buttocks should
still be on your heels. Your hands should be resting beside your body
with your palms facing upwards.*

3

*Relax and breathe into your abdomen. Feel the tension dropping out
from your shoulders onto the floor.*

*This is simple posture can help you connect
to childhood feelings of safety, trust and a
willingness to embrace one's experience.*

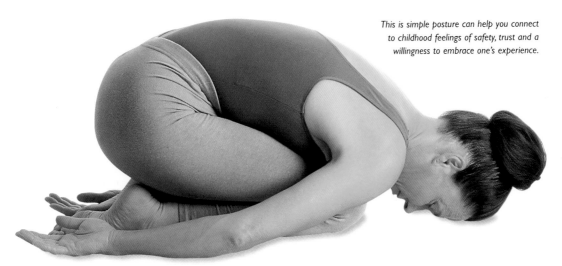

While   you   are   still   seated

Too much time spent sitting in chairs means that many people develop poor posture. The following seated poses work to open up the hips and flex the spine and so can help to counteract long-held bad habits. As with all yoga poses, it is important to move into the postures slowly, working to the capacity of your own body and using your breath and focus to help you deepen and lengthen into each pose.

Bhadrasana –
the Butterfly

While you are doing this exercise, imagine a butterfly gently resting its wings on a lotus leaf. The Butterfly posture opens up the hips, loosens ankles and knees and provides a stretch for the inner thighs.

1

Sit on the floor with your head up and your back straight yet relaxed. Using your hands, bring the soles of your feet together and, holding onto the toes, draw your heels close to your body.

2

Exhale and gently work your thighs down to the floor. Try not to use your elbows to help you by pushing at this stage. Feel a strong stretch on the inner thighs and hips.

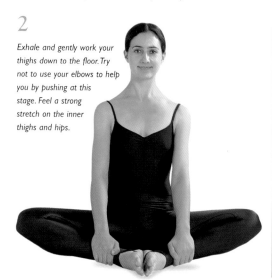

3

Inhale and move the thighs up. As you exhale, move them down again. Repeat about 10 times.

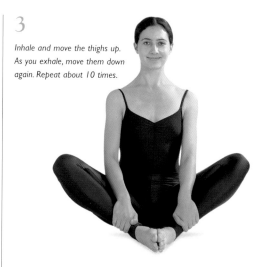

4

Exhale and now you can use your elbows to push your knees and thighs towards the floor. Take your head to meet your toes. Breathe into the position, hold for 10 seconds, then relax.

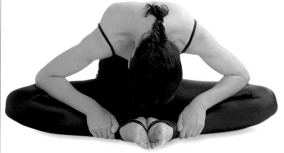

Maricyasana – *the Spinal Twist*

Align your spine, massage the internal organs and force out toxins with the Spinal Twist.

Benefits of Maricyasana

- Tones the liver, spleen and intestines
- Decreases back and hip pain
- Improves the nervous system
- Frees the joints and helps stimulate kundalini energy

1

Sit on the floor with both legs straight in front of you. Bend your right leg and take your right foot outside your left leg. Turn your upper body to the right. Place your left hand near the base of your spine.

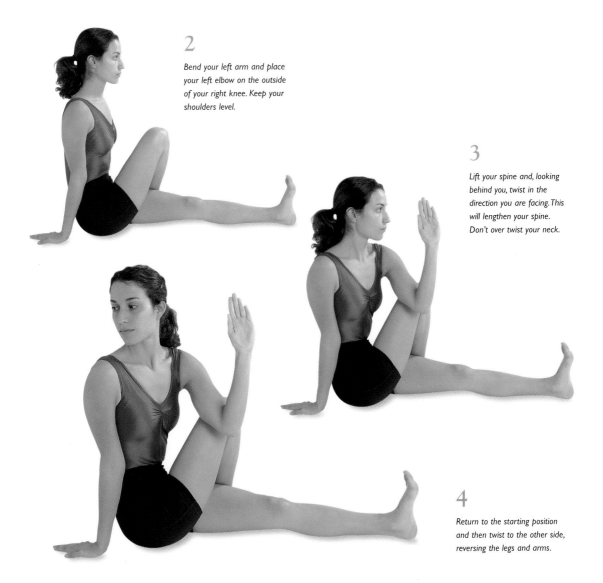

2

Bend your left arm and place your left elbow on the outside of your right knee. Keep your shoulders level.

3

Lift your spine and, looking behind you, twist in the direction you are facing. This will lengthen your spine. Don't over twist your neck.

4

Return to the starting position and then twist to the other side, reversing the legs and arms.

Padmasana – *the Lotus pose*

The lotus flower has its roots in the mud and stretches up through the water to blossom into a beautiful flower, its petals facing the heavens above. Padmasana represents the flower with its leaves open in the light. The Lotus position opens your chest and stimulates the heart chakra. It is revered as a position for meditation and pranayama (see pages 14–17) because it promotes focus.

Caution

Respect the limitations of your body and do not force yourself into this or any other yoga posture. It can be easy to damage the knees in Lotus, which requires flexible hips. Half Lotus (step 2) and Butterfly pose help to open up the hips and you should master these postures before attempting the full Lotus. It can take people many years to master the advanced position of Lotus.

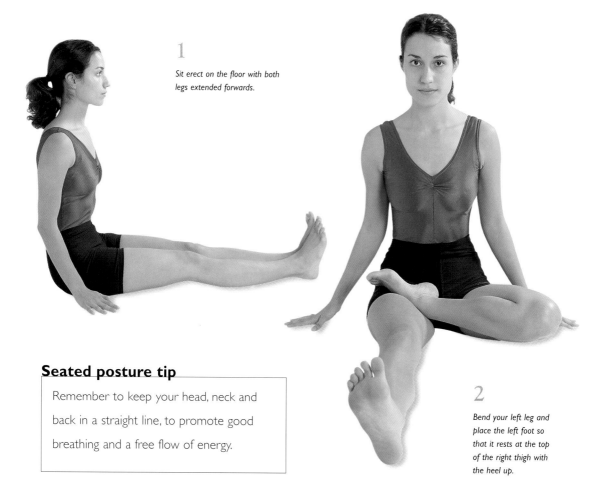

1
Sit erect on the floor with both legs extended forwards.

2
Bend your left leg and place the left foot so that it rests at the top of the right thigh with the heel up.

Seated posture tip

Remember to keep your head, neck and back in a straight line, to promote good breathing and a free flow of energy.

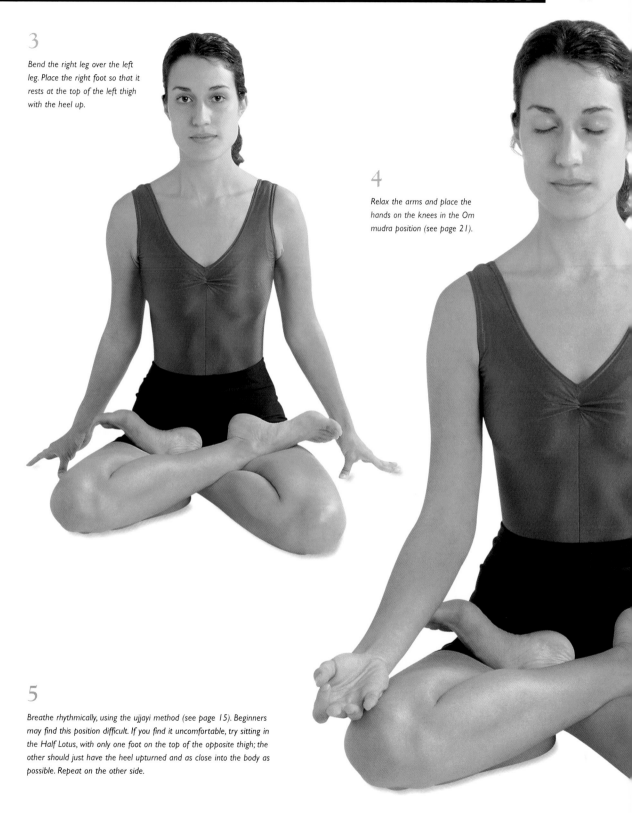

3

Bend the right leg over the left leg. Place the right foot so that it rests at the top of the left thigh with the heel up.

4

Relax the arms and place the hands on the knees in the Om mudra position (see page 21).

5

Breathe rhythmically, using the ujjayi method (see page 15). Beginners may find this position difficult. If you find it uncomfortable, try sitting in the Half Lotus, with only one foot on the top of the opposite thigh; the other should just have the heel upturned and as close into the body as possible. Repeat on the other side.

Improving focus with the balancing postures

Good posture and balance is essential to good health. If your body isn't properly aligned, you will be out of balance; energy will become blocked in certain areas, causing physical and emotional problems. Besides it doesn't look too good either! Yoga will teach you how to get in touch with the poise and strength of your 'inner warrior'.

Vrikshasana — *the Tree*

Practising this asana can bring you a wonderful feeling of inner peace. The balancing postures promote mental concentration, focus and physical balance. For this exercise, visualise yourself as a tree that is firmly rooted to the earth with branches growing up towards the sun. Keep your breathing regular and steady so as not to disturb your balance.

1

Stand straight and get yourself balanced on your left foot. Bend the right knee and place the right foot against the opposite thigh with the knee pointing outwards. Do not lean forwards. The right foot should be flat against the left thigh; the left leg should be straight.

Tip

Focusing on something steady in front of you — such as a fixed point on a wall — can help you to maintain good balance.

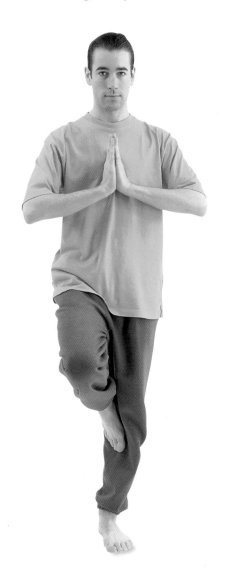

2

Focus on a point in front of you. Now bring both palms together at the chest in Namaste, the prayer position (see page 35). Balance and breathe, using the ujjayi method (see page 15).

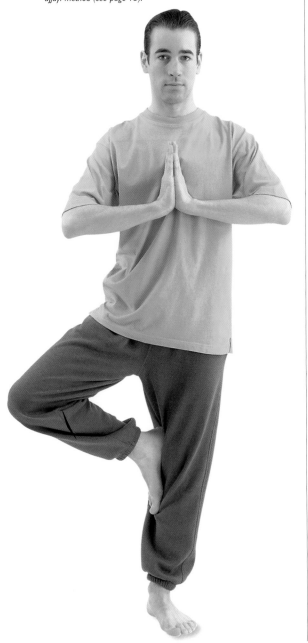

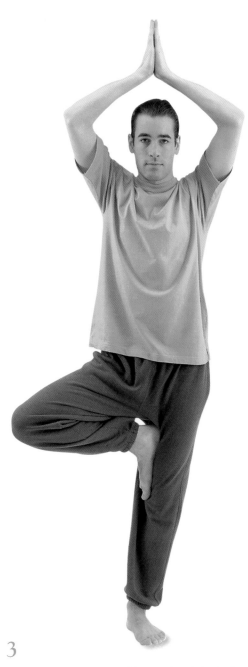

3

Keeping both palms together, extend the arms above the head and stretch to your fingertips. Hold the position for about 30 seconds, breathing gently. Now go back to step 1 and repeat the exercise with the right leg straight and the leftt leg bent. You can gradually increase the time that you hold this posture to a maximum of three minutes.

Natarajasasana – the Cosmic Dancer

The god Shiva as Natarajasasana, the cosmic dancer, destroys and recreates the universe with each step he takes. He destroys the old to make room for the new and symbolises the flow of energy. This posture develops focus and balance and stretches the upper body.

Tips

- Keep the weight firmly on the left leg
- Keep the arm straight, alongside the ear
- Remember to breathe as you hold the pose, keeping your breath steady.

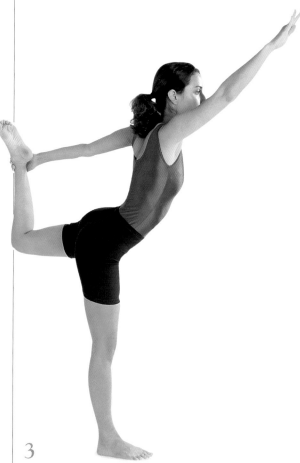

1

Stand with your head and body erect. Bend the left knee and take hold of the ankle behind you with your left hand. Lift the foot up until it is as close to your buttocks as possible. Press down firmly with the right leg and find your point of balance.

2

Inhale and stretch your right arm up straight alongside your right ear. To balance, focus on a point in front of you.

3

Breathe normally and stretch the left foot away from the buttocks behind you, as far back as you can, still keeping hold of the ankle.

4

Focus on a point on the floor just in front of your body. Keeping the right arm alongside your ear, bring the weight of your body forwards until both the chest and the arm are parallel to the floor. Hold the pose for 5–6 breaths and then repeat on the other side.

Squat on Heels and Toes

Although not a classic yoga pose, this exercise helps to improve balance and gives a good stretch to the ankles, heels and foot arches.

1

Stand tall with your feet level and shoulder-width apart. Stretch your arms out straight in front of you and look ahead.

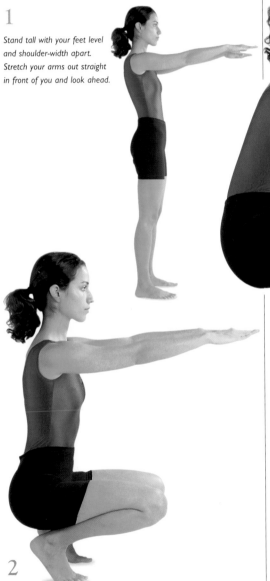

3

Rock back on your heels, come back onto your ankles and stand up straight. Repeat the movement slowly 5–6 times.

Tips

- Make sure you keep your back straight as you squat down onto your toes.

- Keep knees together as you bend.

- Hands and arms should be held straight in front of you throughout the exercise.

2

Keeping your back straight, squat down on your toes, allowing your heels to rise up. Hold the position for a count of two.

Opening the heart and strengthening the back

The back-strengthening postures in this section stretch out the front of the body, open the chest area and strengthen the back of the body. On a subtle level, tightness in the front of the shoulders and the chest indicates a protective psychological mechanism against emotions. The heart chakra is blocked through fear of feeling and energy is unable to flow through freely. When we begin to stretch out and breathe into the chest area with the backbending postures, we open up the heart. While the forward bends are about conquering ego, the backward bends open us up to confronting our fears.

Bhujangasana – *Cobra pose*

The Cobra pose helps to align the spinal disks, strengthen the back and open up the heart chakra. It also energises the nervous system. To perform this exercise, visualise the graceful movement of this powerful and flexible creature. Don't use your arms to support yourself – snakes do not have arms.

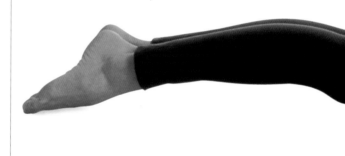

1

Lie on your stomach with your heels and toes together. Place your hands on the floor on either side of your chest, fingers pointing forwards with the tips in line with your shoulders. Your forehead should be on the floor.

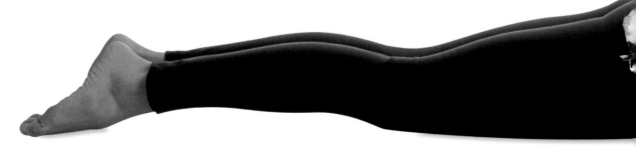

Benefits of Bhujangasana

- Massages and tones all the back muscles

- Expands lungs and chest area

- Helps ease menstrual problems

- Pressure on the abdomen massages all the internal organs

- Increases flexibility of the spine and rejuvenates spinal nerves

- Awakens kundalini energy, the 'coiled serpent' that lies at the base of the spine

2

Inhale, lifting your forehead, chin, shoulders and lastly your chest off the floor. Keep the hips pressed down to the floor. Elbows should be slightly bent and shoulders relaxed. Roll the body up and back. Breathe and hold the position for 10–15 seconds, then relax back to the floor.

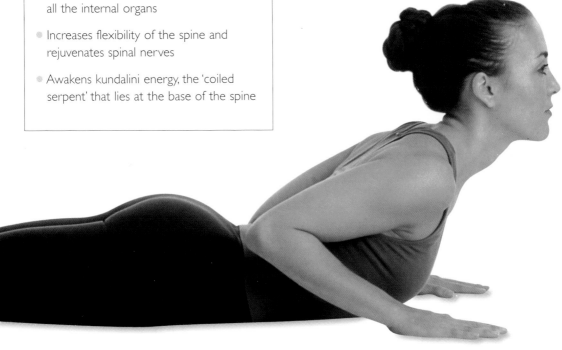

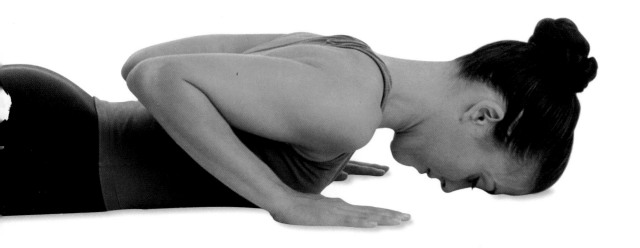

Dhanurasana – the Bow

For this exercise, imagine your body as an archer's bow about to launch an arrow. This is a high-energy posture that massages the back, tones the stomach, improves concentration and keeps the spine supple. Regular practice of this asana promotes energy and vitality.

The Bow

It is important to keep your arms and elbows straight in this pose. Your shoulders should be pressed down and back.

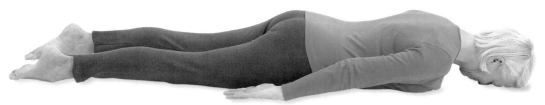

1

Lie on your front with your body straight, your arms by your sides and your forehead resting gently on the ground.

2

Bend the knees and bring the feet up. Reach back with the hands to hold the ankles. Inhale and bring your feet as high as you can, keeping them away from your body.

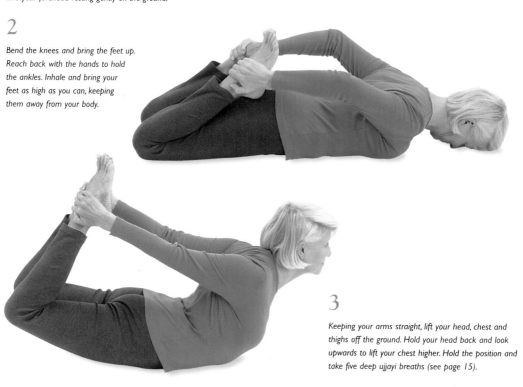

3

Keeping your arms straight, lift your head, chest and thighs off the ground. Hold your head back and look upwards to lift your chest higher. Hold the position and take five deep ujjayi breaths (see page 15).

Salabhasana – *the Locust posture*

This is an exercise that helps in the development of the cardiac muscles while strengthening the lower extremity of the spine. It promotes digestion and also tones the muscles of the bladder.

Tips

- The shoulders and chin should remain in contact with the floor

- Avoid the tendency to twist the hips

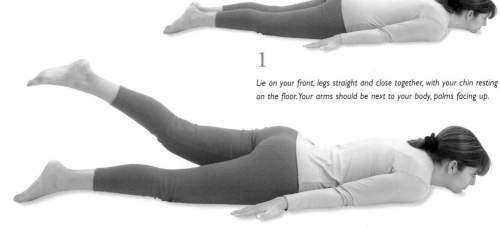

1

Lie on your front, legs straight and close together, with your chin resting on the floor. Your arms should be next to your body, palms facing up.

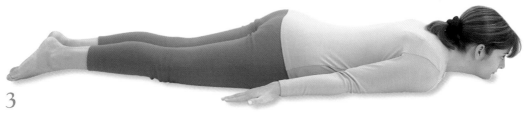

2

Inhale and raise up your left leg to an angle of 45 degrees. Keep your legs straight, toes pointed. Hold the position for two breaths.

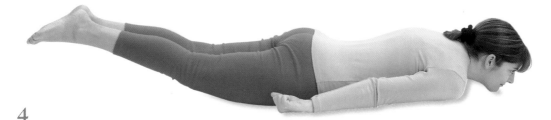

3

Exhale and gently lower your leg. Inhale and repeat on the right leg, again holding the position for two breaths.

4

Inhale, and this time raise up both legs to an angle of 45 degrees. Again keep your legs straight, together and with toes pointed. Hold the posture for five ujjayi breaths (see page 15). Exhale and lower your legs. Relax.

Ustrasana — the Camel

The Camel works on opening up the chest and releasing the shoulders. You should feel a strong stretch to the thighs, abdomen and the rib muscles. This pose can also help people who are suffering from sciatica — inflammation of the sciatic nerve that runs from the hip down the back of the leg.

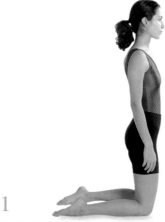

1

Kneel on the floor with your feet slightly apart behind you and your back, neck and head forming a straight line.

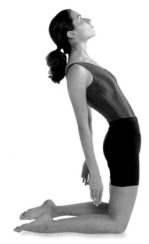

2

Stretch your hips and thighs forwards and reach your arms back towards your heels. Visualise your thighs pressed up against a wall in front of you. Your spine extends upwards as you lean back.

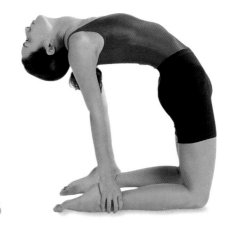

3

As you bend backwards, try to catch hold of your heels with your hands. Tilt your head backwards and look up.

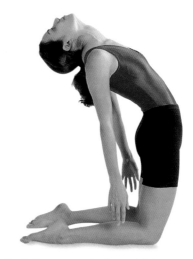

4

Hold the position for five steady breaths. On an exhalation, come up slowly, preventing your spine from twisting as you do.

Tip

If you find that you can't grasp your heels to begin with, keep your hands on your hips when you lean back. Eventually you will be able to reach your heels, but be patient with yourself. Strength comes with practice.

Matsyasana – *the Fish*

The Fish stretches the spine and at the same time expands and opens the chest. The most important benefit of this posture is the regulation of the four parathyroid glands in the neck. These endocrine glands control the levels of calcium in the blood. Calcium, as we all know, strengthens bones and teeth. It is also important for the contraction of muscles and the clotting of blood.

Benefits of Matsyasana

- Corrects rounded shoulders
- Increases lung capacity and helps with breathing problems
- Relieves stress and regulates moods
- Increases prana in the neck, shoulders, lungs, stomach and spleen
- Energises the parathyroid glands and tones the pituitary

1

Lie flat on your back, with your legs together and your knees straight. Place your arms under your thighs with your palms facing downwards.

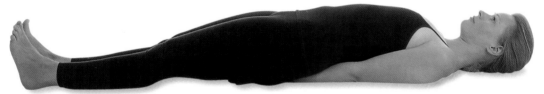

2

Bend your elbows and push them into the floor. Lift your chest upwards but make sure that your legs and buttocks remain on the floor.

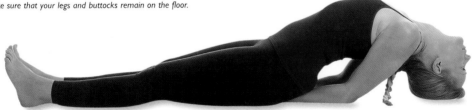

3

Take your head back and rest the top of your head on the floor, with your chest wide open. Keep your weight on your elbows. Breathe into your chest and abdomen. Hold the position for 10–20 seconds. As you gain strength, try holding it for a little longer each time.

Tips

- Check your weight is on your elbows and that they are not sticking out.
- Arch up your chest as high as possible.

The inverted postures

It is important to end a yoga session with inverted postures. They help to quieten the mind in preparation for relaxation and cool down the body. Blood flows more easily to the upper body, heart and brain, helping to improve the circulation and combat lethargy. Being upside-down also helps to give you a different view of the world.

Sarvangasana – the Shoulderstand

This is an inverted posture that will invigorate and rejuvenate the whole of your body. Its most important function, however, is to stimulate the thyroid and parathyroid glands as the chin is pressed into the base of the throat. Since it limits the use of the top of the lungs, it encourages deep abdominal breathing and can promote patience, relaxation and a feeling of letting go. You can practise the shoulderstand for many minutes.

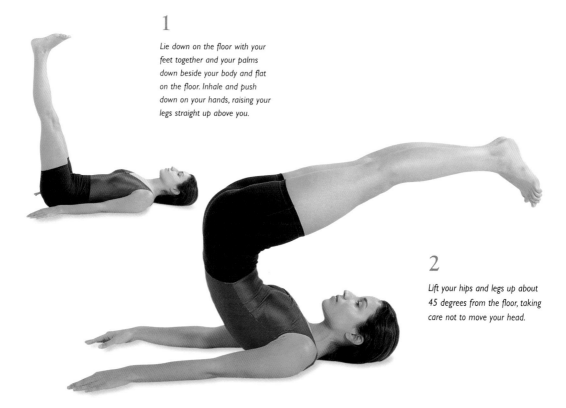

1

Lie down on the floor with your feet together and your palms down beside your body and flat on the floor. Inhale and push down on your hands, raising your legs straight up above you.

2

Lift your hips and legs up about 45 degrees from the floor, taking care not to move your head.

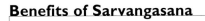

Benefits of Sarvangasana

- Stretches the spine, helping to keep it strong and supple

- Regulates the thyroid and the parathyroid glands

- Helps venous blood to flow to the heart, thereby relieving varicose veins

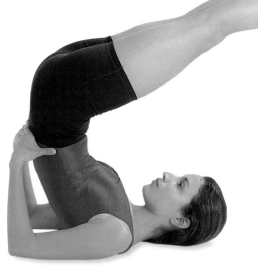

3

Exhale and support your back with your hands, keeping your arms as close to your shoulders as possible. Thumbs are around the front of your body, fingers at the back. Lift your legs up.

Caution

Do not perform the Shoulderstand if you:

- suffer from high blood pressure

- have any eye problems

- are very overweight

- are menstruating or pregnant

4

Straighten your back and take your legs up to a vertical position. Breathe into the posture, keeping as straight as possible by pulling in your buttocks. Keep your arms close to your body with your hands near your shoulders. Your feet should be relaxed and pointing towards the ceiling. Hold the position for five ujjayi breaths (see page 15).

Halasana – *the Plough*

Beginning from Shoulderstand (see page 54), the Plough is an extreme forward bend promoting strength and flexibility to the back and neck. Breathe rhythmically and make sure you don't twist your head or neck.

Benefits of Halasana

- Strengthens the nervous system
- Improves blood circulation
- Stimulates and massages internal organs
- Releases any tension from the shoulders and upper back region
- Decreases insomnia

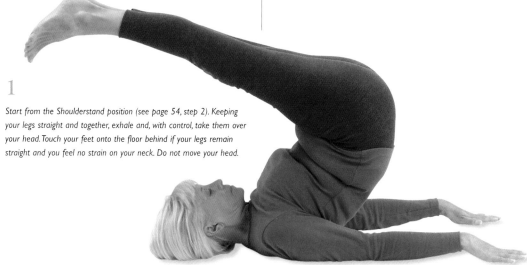

1

Start from the Shoulderstand position (see page 54, step 2). Keeping your legs straight and together, exhale and, with control, take them over your head. Touch your feet onto the floor behind if your legs remain straight and you feel no strain on your neck. Do not move your head.

2

If your feet can reach, place your hands, palms down, behind your head. Push your heels to the floor with your toes tucked in towards your body. Press the toes firmly down, lifting your hips to give a stretch to the hamstrings. Hold the pose for about a minute. As you become stronger, you can hold the position for a longer period.

Setu Bandha Sarvangasana – *the Bridge*

This position counterposes the previous two postures, helping to release any tension that may have built up. The Bridge helps to strengthen the neck and spine and also increases your lung capacity.

1

Lie flat on the floor on your back with your knees bent and shoulder-width apart. Your arms should be alongside your body.

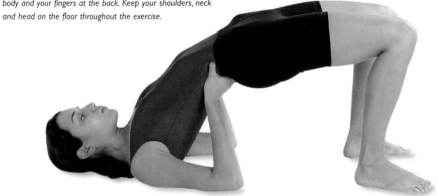

2

Exhale and raise your hips, supporting your lower back with your hands. Your thumbs should be around the front of your body and your fingers at the back. Keep your shoulders, neck and head on the floor throughout the exercise.

3

Lift your hips and chest as high up as possible and breathe into the chest. You should feel a good stretch on your thighs. Keep your knees parallel with your toes pointing forwards. Try to keep your neck, head and shoulders on the floor, and breathe deeply into the chest rather than the abdomen. Hold the position for five ujjayi breaths (see page 15).

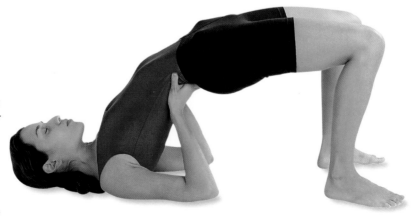

Sirshasana – the Headstand

This king/queen of postures stimulates the entire system; it improves circulation, nourishes the spinal column, nervous system and brain, increases memory and focus and enhances breathing. For the Headstand, you need sufficient strength in your arms, stomach, shoulders and neck, which can be developed through regular practice of standing postures.

Caution

- Practise the headstand with a wall behind you in case you lose balance. You should not attempt it if you:

- suffer from high blood pressure

- have any eye problems

- are very overweight

- are menstruating or pregnant

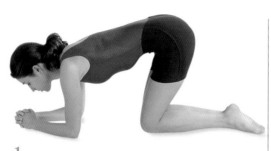

1

Begin from Child's pose (see page 39). Sit back. Keep the elbows on the floor and clasp each with the opposite hand. Release the hands and interlink the fingers in front of you, making a tripod of elbows and hands.

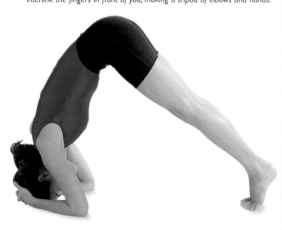

2

Place the back of your head firmly against your clasped hands. Now straighten your legs, raising your hips upwards. Push down on your elbows. Your body should take the form of an inverted 'V' shape.

3

Walk the feet towards the elbows and feel your back straighten until the hips are over the head. Bend your knees and lift the feet off the ground, bringing heels to the buttocks. Keep your weight on the elbows, not the head.

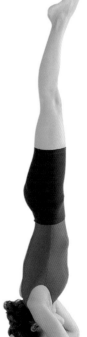

4

Slowly start to straighten your knees, taking your feet up to the ceiling. Try to hold this position for 30 seconds, breathing normally. You can gradually increase it to 3 minutes. Come down by bending your knees, then the hips and with control take the feet down to the floor. Now relax in the Child's pose (see page 39).

Kakasana – *the Crow*

Like the Tree (see pages 44–45), the Crow is a good exercise for improving physical and mental balance. It's fun to practise but requires focus. It may look advanced, but it is relatively easy to perform once you get your balance.

The posture will develop strength in the upper body, but the trick lies in keeping your balance as you transfer your weight onto your hands. Ensure your hips are raised, your knees resting on the upper arms and your head up. Your feet should be together and relaxed.

Benefits of Kakasana

- Stretches out the arms, wrists and shoulders, increasing flexibility

- Strengthens the arms, shoulders, wrists and hands

- Increases breathing capacity

- Develops mental focus and your powers of concentration

- Improves awareness and mental poise

- Promotes inner balance and improves vitality and energy

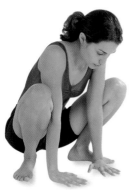

1

From a squatting position, place your palms firmly on the floor. They should be directly under your shoulders and between your knees. Spread your fingers (like the feet of a crow).

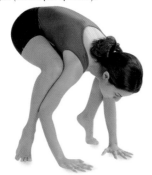

2

Bend your elbows outwards, rise up on your toes and rest your knees on your outspread upper arms. Inhale, retain your breath and gradually transfer your weight forwards and onto your outspread hands.

3

Slowly lift your feet, gradually bringing the full weight of your body onto your hands. Breathe steadily and hold the position for as long as is possible.

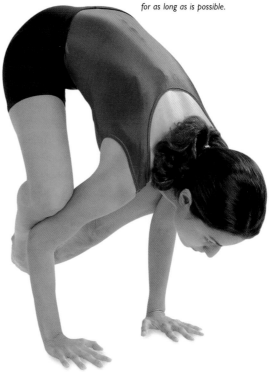

Be mindful with
your thoughts

Our thoughts and beliefs serve to create our reality. Because of this, changing our thoughts can change our lives. You could say thinking is a serious responsibility. Giving any thought our attention will help it to grow. A negative thought will grow as much as a positive one and will affect our experience of life accordingly.

The basic component of our physical universe is energy. Matter is composed of dense energy; thoughts are composed of finer energy. Whatever we create, we create in thought form first. The thought creates an image, a form, which magnetises energy to flow into the image and eventually manifest itself on the physical plane. We will create, and therefore attract into our lives the beliefs and desires that we focus on the most intensely. If we are negative and fearful, we will attract experiences into our lives that echo those thoughts and feelings. When we are positive in attitude, we attract more pleasure, good health and happiness into our lives.

The practice of yoga is one that fully embraces positive thinking as one of its most important principles. It helps us to discard old thoughts, beliefs and attitudes that no longer support us. It connects us to the intelligence and wisdom of our bodies and helps us to use the power of our minds constructively.

Our successes and failures are not caused by 'the world out there', but by our inner world. By exploring our inner world and bringing it into consciousness, we can understand the hidden agendas through which we create our reality. We don't have to spend years in psychoanalysis to 'find ourselves'. We can relax and enjoy the process through yoga, 'the ancient science of life'.

Yoga gives us an opportunity to hear the wisdom of our body, find the stillness of our mind and create a happier way of being.

Working creatively with your thoughts

To work creatively with your thoughts, you need to learn to control them. You can do this by learning to still the reactive mind and release it from negative conditioning and old patterns of behaviour that no longer serve you. Meditation, mantras, affirmations, breath control and visualisation all serve as tools to help you.

Meditation is the tool for cleansing the mind of limitations and fears, releasing creative energy and finding peace by connecting the personal self with the universal self. In order to meditate, it is important to develop powers of concentration. Mantras, affirmations and breath control will help you to develop focus.

Affirmations are positively stated words repeated over and over to reprogramme the subconscious. You need to think very carefully about the qualities you want to acquire in yourself and state them in the present tense. The subconscious mind will respond to exactly what you tell it. If, for example, you say: 'I am going to be fit and healthy', it puts it in the future so the mind will respond to 'going to be' and not to 'being'. If you say 'I am fit and healthy', your power is in the present.

Mantras are sounds that resonate in the body evoking certain energies. Gradually the chanting of mantras will produce an altered state of consciousness. You can begin by constantly repeating the mantra verbally and later mentally. Alternatively, you can meditate by concentrating on the sound of your breath and detaching your mind from the thoughts that pass through. Once you are sitting in a comfortable position with your back straight, you can begin to relax by breathing rhythmically. Let go and enjoy the feeling. Now choose a mantra or affirmation and repeat it again and again mentally, or focus on an image. It can be a flower, colour, or any image. When your mind starts to wander, guide it back to the object of focus. It may take quite a while to develop concentration, but continue the practice even if it is only for a few minutes a day. Gradually, as your concentration improves, your time spent in meditation will lengthen. If you can't think of a suitable mantra, try repeating this one: Om Shanti Shanti Shanti – Peace, Peace, Peace. Enjoy your journey!

Glossary

Adho Mukha Shvanasana
Downward-facing Dog;
a forward bend.

Ajna chakra
The sixth chakra, located at
the 'third eye', the point
between the eyebrows.

Anahata chakra
The fourth chakra, located at
the heart centre.

Anuloma Viloma
Alternate nostril breathing.

Asana
Physical yogic exercise. Asana
is a Sanskrit word that
translates as 'posture'.

Astral body
The subtle body containing the
prana, emotions and the mind.

Aswini mudra
A lock that strengthens the
pelvic muscles.

Bhadrasana
The Butterfly pose.

Bhujangasana
The Cobra; a backbend.

Bilikasana
The Cat pose.

Chakras
Energy centres in the
ethereal astral body.

Dhanurasana
The Bow; a backbend.

Gunas
These are the three qualities
of nature: Sattva, Rajas and
Tamas. Everything in the
universe is made up of gunas,
in different proportions.

Halasana
The Sanskrit name for the
Plough, an inverted posture.

Hatha yoga
The path of yoga that deals
primarily with the physical
body as the path to
enlightenment.

Ida
One of the three main
meridians in the astral body
through which prana, or
energy, passes. Located to the
left of the sushumna.

Janu Shirshanasana
Sitting One Leg; a forward
bend posture.

Kakasana
The Sanskrit name for the
Crow; a balancing posture.

Kapalabhati
A cleansing exercise to clear
the lungs, sinuses and
respiratory tract.

Kundalini
The cosmic energy that
resides in the base chakra.

Manipura chakra
The third chakra,
corresponding to the solar
plexus and the main
storehouse for prana.

Mantra
A magical word or phrase
repeated either verbally or
mentally. It is used to focus
the mind during meditation.

Maricyasana
The Half Spinal Twist; a
twisting position.

Matsyasana
The Fish pose; a back-
bending exercise.

Mudhasana
The Pose of the Child; a
forward bend.

Mudra
A hand position or yoga 'seal'
that channels prana.

Muladhara chakra
The lowest chakra, located at
the base of the spine.

Nadis
The subtle channels in the
astral body through which
prana can flow.

Namaste mudra
A mudra in which the hands are placed together in the prayer position.

OM
Pronounced A-U-M – the sacred symbol of God as the absolute; a mudra used during meditation – the sound of the universe's vibration.

Padma Shirasana
The Lotus pose; a meditative posture which is said to resemble the lotus flower.

Parsvottanasana
The Side Angle stretch; a standing posture.

Pingala
Located on the right of the sushumna and one of the three most important nadis for channelling prana in the astral body.

Prana
The life force that flows through the nadis of the astral body.

Pranayama
Breathing exercises for purifying and strengthening the mind and body.

Rajas
One of the three gunas, rasa has the qualities of overactivity and passion.

Sahasrara chakra
The seventh and highest chakra; it is located at the crown of the head

Sanskrit
The most ancient literary language of India, said to be the language of the gods.

Sarvangasana
The Shoulderstand; an inverted posture.

Sattva
One of the three gunas, sattva has the qualities of purity and lightness.

Savasana
The Corpse pose; a relaxation posture.

Setu Bandha Sarvangasana
The Bridge pose; a back-bending posture.

Shakti
The primordial cosmic energy seen in the personification of the Great Goddess, or kundalini.

Siva
Hindu god and the divine inspiration of yoga.

Surya Namaskara
The Sun Salutations.

Sushumna
A channel in the astral body corresponding to the spine and through which kundalini energy can travel.

Swadhishtana chakra
The second chakra; situated in the genital region.

Tadasana
The Mountain pose; a standing posture.

Tamas
A guna with the qualities of inertia, lethargy and laziness.

Trikonasana
The Sanskrit name for the Triangle; a standing posture.

Ujjayi
A breathing technique that produces a throaty sound.

Uttanasana
Standing Head to Knee; a forward bend.

Virabhadrasana
The Warrior; a standing pose.

Vishuddha chakra
The fifth energy centre in the astral body; it is located at the base of the throat.

Yoga mudra
A forward bend.

Yogi
A male who practises yoga.

Yogini
A female who practises yoga.

Index